LYMPHATIC MASSAGE LUMINESCENCE

The Glow Getter's Guide to Effortless Radiance With Lymphatic Drainage Massage for perfect skin glow

Melissa O'Brian

INTRODUCTION

The introduction sets the stage for the entire book, providing readers with essential background information on lymphatic drainage massage and its impact on skin health.

Understanding the Lymphatic System

The lymphatic system is a crucial part of the body's circulatory and immune systems. It consists of lymph nodes, vessels, and organs that work together to transport lymph – a clear fluid containing white blood cells – throughout the body. This system plays a pivotal role in filtering toxins, waste, and excess fluids from the tissues, supporting immune function, and maintaining fluid balance.

Understanding the intricate network of lymphatic vessels and nodes is fundamental to grasping the significance of lymphatic drainage massage. When the lymphatic system is compromised or sluggish, it can lead to fluid retention, impaired immune function, and dull, congested skin. By delving into the anatomy and physiology of the lymphatic system, readers can gain a deeper appreciation for the targeted benefits that lymphatic drainage massage can offer.

Benefits of Lymphatic Drainage Massage for Skin

Lymphatic drainage massage is renowned for its transformative effects on the skin. As the lymphatic system plays a vital role in eliminating waste and supporting overall health, its impact on skin appearance is profound. The benefits extend beyond mere aesthetics, reaching into the realms of holistic well-being.

One primary benefit is the reduction of puffiness and swelling. Lymphatic drainage massage facilitates the removal of excess fluid and toxins, diminishing the appearance of bloated or swollen skin. This is particularly beneficial for individuals struggling with facial puffiness or under-eye bags.

Improving circulation is another key advantage. By enhancing lymphatic flow, the massage encourages better blood circulation, delivering oxygen and nutrients to the skin cells. This improved blood flow contributes to a healthier complexion, promoting a natural glow and radiance.

Furthermore, lymphatic drainage massage can aid in detoxification. By expelling toxins and waste through the lymphatic system, the skin is relieved of the burden of processing and eliminating these substances. This detoxifying effect can lead to clearer, more vibrant skin.

The massage also promotes relaxation, which has indirect yet significant benefits for the skin. Stress and tension can manifest on the skin's surface, contributing to issues like acne and premature aging. Lymphatic drainage massage helps alleviate stress, fostering a calm and serene state that reflects positively on the skin.

In essence, the benefits of lymphatic drainage massage for the skin encompass both physical and emotional aspects. By understanding and harnessing the power of this therapeutic technique, individuals can unlock the potential for healthier, more radiant skin, creating a harmonious connection between internal well-being and external beauty.

1

THE BASICS OF LYMPHATIC DRAINAGE MASSAGE

Lymphatic drainage massage is a specialized technique designed to enhance the flow of lymphatic fluid throughout the body, promoting optimal function of the lymphatic system. This section will explore the fundamental aspects of this massage therapy, focusing on techniques and movements that define its efficacy.

Techniques and Movements

Lymphatic drainage massage employs gentle, rhythmic movements that aim to stimulate the lymphatic vessels and nodes. The techniques used are distinct from traditional massage, as the emphasis is on light pressure and specific directional strokes.

One primary technique is manual lymphatic drainage (MLD), which involves gentle, circular motions and pumping movements. These techniques encourage the movement of lymph towards the lymph nodes, where waste products can be filtered and eliminated from the body. Practitioners often use their hands, fingers, or specialized tools to perform these precise and targeted maneuvers.

Another essential aspect of lymphatic drainage massage is the sequence of movements. Therapists follow a specific order, starting from the areas with the most significant lymphatic concentration, typically the neck and face, and gradually progressing to other parts of the body. This systematic approach ensures thorough lymphatic stimulation and effective waste removal.

In addition to manual techniques, practitioners may incorporate other modalities such as cupping or vibration to enhance lymphatic flow. These techniques, when applied skillfully, can amplify the benefits of lymphatic drainage massage, contributing to improved skin health and overall well-being.

Contraindications and Precautions

While lymphatic drainage massage is generally safe and well-tolerated, there are specific contraindications and precautions that practitioners must consider to ensure the safety of the client. Understanding these factors is crucial for both therapists and individuals seeking this type of massage.

Contraindications refer to situations where the massage should not be performed, as it may pose risks or exacerbate existing conditions. Some contraindications for lymphatic drainage massage include acute infections, such as cellulitis, as the massage could potentially spread the infection. Additionally, individuals with congestive heart failure or active cancer may need to avoid lymphatic drainage massage, as it can affect fluid balance and the lymphatic system's workload.

Precautions, on the other hand, highlight circumstances where the massage can be performed with adjustments or additional considerations. For example, caution should be exercised when working with clients who have a history of deep vein thrombosis (DVT) or thrombophlebitis, as the massage could potentially dislodge blood clots. In such cases, therapists may need to modify techniques or focus on areas away from the affected area.

Pregnancy is another scenario that requires special attention. While lymphatic drainage massage can be beneficial for reducing swelling and promoting relaxation during pregnancy, therapists must be trained in prenatal massage techniques and take precautions to ensure the safety of both the mother and the baby.

Understanding these contraindications and precautions is essential for responsible and effective practice. Before undergoing lymphatic drainage massage, individuals should communicate openly with their therapists about any pre-existing conditions, medications, or concerns to ensure a safe and tailored experience. This attention to safety contributes to the overall positive outcomes and experiences associated with lymphatic drainage massage.

2

HOW THE LYMPHATIC SYSTEM AFFECTS SKIN HEALTH

Understanding the intricate relationship between the lymphatic system and skin health is key to appreciating the significance of incorporating lymphatic drainage massage into skincare routines. This section will delve into the physiological connections and the profound impact the lymphatic system has on the skin.

Relationship between Lymphatic System and Skin

The relationship between the lymphatic system and the skin is symbiotic, playing a vital role in maintaining overall health and well-being. The skin, being the largest organ of the body, serves as a protective barrier against external threats, while the lymphatic system acts as a filtration and drainage system, ensuring the removal of waste and toxins.

The lymphatic vessels, intertwined with the skin's connective tissues, play a crucial role in regulating fluid balance. They transport lymph – a clear fluid containing immune cells, waste products, and excess fluids – away from the tissues and towards the lymph nodes. Here, harmful substances are filtered out, and the cleansed lymph is returned to the bloodstream.

When the lymphatic system functions optimally, the skin reaps numerous benefits. Efficient drainage helps prevent fluid retention, reducing the risk of puffiness and swelling. This is particularly noticeable in facial tissues, where poor lymphatic circulation can contribute to a tired or bloated appearance.

Furthermore, the lymphatic system is closely linked to the immune response. Lymph nodes, often found near the surface of the skin, act as crucial hubs for immune cells. A well-functioning lymphatic system helps bolster the skin's defenses, aiding in the rapid identification and elimination of pathogens.

Impact on Radiance and Glow

The impact of the lymphatic system on skin radiance and glow is profound. One of the primary contributors to a lackluster complexion is the accumulation of toxins and waste products in the skin tissues. When the lymphatic system becomes sluggish or overloaded, the skin's ability to detoxify is compromised, leading to a dull and fatigued appearance.

Lymphatic drainage massage emerges as a powerful ally in restoring skin radiance. By employing gentle, targeted techniques, this massage stimulates lymphatic circulation, facilitating the removal of accumulated waste. As toxins are flushed away, the skin is rejuvenated, and its natural luminosity is restored.

Improved circulation is another mechanism through which the lymphatic system enhances skin glow. The lymphatic vessels work in tandem with blood vessels to nourish the skin cells. When lymphatic flow is enhanced, blood circulation improves as well, ensuring a robust supply of oxygen and nutrients to the skin. This heightened nutrient exchange contributes to a healthier complexion, marked by a youthful radiance.

The reduction of puffiness and swelling achieved through lymphatic drainage massage also contributes to a more vibrant appearance. Facial puffiness, often associated with fluid retention, can obscure the contours of the face and create shadows, making the skin appear less vibrant. By promoting the efficient drainage of excess fluid, the massage helps sculpt facial features, unveiling a more defined and radiant visage.

The impact on skin glow is not only superficial but extends to deeper layers. A well-functioning lymphatic system supports the overall health of skin cells, promoting optimal regeneration and repair. This cellular resilience translates into a skin that not only looks radiant but also feels resilient and revitalized.

In essence, the relationship between the lymphatic system and skin health is a dynamic interplay that goes beyond surface aesthetics. By nurturing the lymphatic system through practices like lymphatic drainage massage, individuals can unlock the key to a luminous and vibrant complexion that reflects the harmonious balance of internal well-being and external beauty.

3

PREPARING FOR A LYMPHATIC DRAINAGE MASSAGE

Preparation is a crucial aspect of ensuring a successful and enjoyable lymphatic drainage massage experience. This section will explore the key components of preparing for this specialized massage therapy, including client assessment and creating a relaxing environment.

Client Assessment

A thorough client assessment is the foundation upon which an effective lymphatic drainage massage session is built. This process involves gathering essential information about the client's health, lifestyle, and specific concerns to tailor the massage to their unique needs.

The assessment typically begins with a detailed consultation. During this discussion, the therapist gathers information about the client's medical history, including any existing health conditions, surgeries, or medications. Understanding the client's health status is crucial, as certain conditions may require modifications to the massage techniques or, in some cases, contraindicate the treatment altogether.

In addition to medical history, the therapist may inquire about the client's lifestyle factors, such as diet, hydration, and exercise habits. These factors can significantly influence the lymphatic system's function and overall well-being. For example, dehydration or a diet high in sodium may contribute to fluid retention, impacting the effectiveness of the massage.

Aesthetic concerns are also addressed during the assessment. Clients may express specific skin issues or cosmetic goals they hope to achieve through lymphatic drainage massage. Whether it's reducing puffiness, improving skin texture, or enhancing radiance, understanding these objectives allows the therapist to customize the massage techniques and focus areas accordingly.

Beyond verbal communication, physical assessments may be conducted to evaluate the client's lymphatic circulation and identify areas of congestion or swelling. This hands-on evaluation helps the therapist tailor the massage to address specific concerns and ensures a personalized and effective session.

Overall, client assessment sets the stage for a safe and customized lymphatic drainage massage. By gathering comprehensive information, therapists can adapt their approach to meet individual needs, providing a more targeted and beneficial experience for the client.

Creating a Relaxing Environment

The ambiance in which a lymphatic drainage massage takes place significantly influences the overall experience and effectiveness of the treatment. Creating a relaxing environment is essential to help clients unwind, release tension, and maximize the therapeutic benefits of the massage.

Lighting and Atmosphere:

Begin by considering the lighting in the massage room. Soft, diffused lighting creates a calming ambiance. Consider using dimmable lights or candles to adjust the intensity based on the client's preference. The overall atmosphere should be tranquil, providing a refuge from daily stressors.

Music and Soundscapes:

Selecting soothing music or nature sounds can enhance the relaxation experience. Calming instrumental music or gentle ocean waves create an auditory backdrop that complements the massage. Ensure that the volume is adjustable to cater to individual preferences.

Temperature Control:

Maintaining a comfortable room temperature is crucial for relaxation. Clients should be able to easily adjust the temperature to their liking. Providing blankets or heated massage tables adds an extra layer of comfort, promoting a cozy and nurturing environment.

Aromatherapy:

Incorporating aromatherapy can elevate the sensory experience. Essential oils such as lavender, chamomile, or eucalyptus are known for their relaxation-inducing properties. Ensure that the chosen scents align with any potential sensitivities or preferences the client may have.

Clean and Tidy Space:

A clutter-free and well-organized massage room contributes to a sense of tranquility. Ensure that all necessary supplies are within easy reach, and the massage table is properly draped and cushioned for comfort.

Communication and Comfort:

Establishing clear communication with the client before the session ensures that their preferences and concerns are considered. Inquire about any specific areas of discomfort or sensitivity. Provide a comfortable robe or disposable undergarments for the client to wear during the massage.

Privacy and Disconnect:

Encourage clients to disconnect from electronic devices before the session to fully immerse themselves in the experience. Privacy is essential, so ensure that the massage room provides a secure and intimate space for the client to relax without external disturbances.

By meticulously curating a serene and welcoming environment, therapists enhance the overall impact of lymphatic drainage massage. A relaxed atmosphere not only contributes to the physical benefits of the massage but also fosters a mental and emotional sense of well-being. This holistic approach ensures that clients leave not only with improved skin health but also with a renewed sense of calm and balance.

4

STEP-BY-STEP GUIDE TO LYMPHATIC DRAINAGE MASSAGE

Lymphatic drainage massage is a precise and targeted technique that requires a systematic approach to ensure optimal results. This section will provide a detailed step-by-step guide for both face and neck techniques, as well as body techniques, outlining the key movements and considerations for an effective lymphatic drainage massage.

Face and Neck Techniques

1. Start with Neck Draining:

Begin the massage by gently draining the lymph nodes in the neck. Use light, sweeping motions with your fingertips, moving from the base of the neck towards the collarbone. This helps open up the lymphatic vessels and prepares the area for more focused techniques.

2. Address the Jawline:

Using upward strokes, massage the jawline to encourage lymphatic flow. Pay attention to the space behind the ears, as lymph nodes in this area play a crucial role in facial drainage. Use gentle, circular motions to stimulate this region.

3. Focus on the Cheeks:

Move to the cheeks, employing light, sweeping motions towards the ears. The goal is to guide the lymphatic fluid towards the lymph nodes. Be mindful of the delicate skin on the face, adjusting pressure accordingly.

4. Under-Eye Drainage:

Reduce puffiness and address under-eye bags by using gentle tapping or pulsing motions with your fingertips. Start from the inner corners of the eyes and move towards the temples. This technique promotes drainage in the eye area, minimizing fluid retention.

5. Nasolabial Fold and Mouth Area:

Address the nasolabial fold (the lines from the nose to the mouth) and the mouth area with upward and outward strokes. Focus on guiding the lymphatic fluid towards the outer edges of the face.

6. Forehead and Scalp Massage:

Conclude the face and neck massage by gently working on the forehead and scalp. Use circular motions to cover the entire forehead and finish with light, sweeping movements through the hair. This helps release tension and encourages lymphatic drainage.

Body Techniques

1. Start at the Collarbone:

For the body, initiate the massage by gently stimulating the lymph nodes near the collarbone. Use light, upward strokes to encourage the flow of lymphatic fluid towards these central nodes.

2. Arm and Hand Massage:

Move to the arms, employing long, sweeping strokes towards the armpits. Pay attention to the inner elbow and wrist areas. Continue down to the hands, using circular motions to address each finger. This technique helps reduce swelling and promotes fluid circulation.

3. Upper Body Draining:

Focus on the upper body, using gentle strokes from the chest towards the armpits. This technique targets the lymph nodes in the chest and underarms, facilitating the drainage of toxins and waste.

4. Abdominal Massage:

Perform light, circular movements on the abdomen. Start clockwise, following the natural flow of the intestines. This aids in digestive function and encourages lymphatic drainage in the abdominal area.

5. Leg and Foot Massage:

Move to the legs, using upward strokes towards the groin area. Pay attention to the inner thigh and knee areas. Continue down to the feet, employing circular motions on the soles and gentle stretching of the toes. This technique is effective in reducing fluid retention in the lower extremities.

6. Final Full-Body Strokes:

Conclude the body massage with full-body strokes. Use long, sweeping motions from the extremities towards the central areas of the body. This helps integrate the lymphatic drainage throughout the entire system.

Considerations for Both Face and Body Techniques:

- Consistent Pressure:

Maintain a consistent, gentle pressure throughout the massage. The goal is to encourage lymphatic flow without causing discomfort or irritation to the skin.

- Directional Movements:

Always move in the direction of lymphatic flow. This typically means moving towards the central lymph nodes – the collarbone for the upper body and the groin area for the lower body.

- Customization for Individual Needs:

Tailor the massage to address specific concerns or areas of focus. If a client has particular areas of congestion or puffiness, allocate more time and attention to those regions.

- Hydration:

Encourage clients to stay hydrated before and after the massage. Hydration supports the lymphatic system's function and enhances the effectiveness of the massage.

- Post-Massage Care:

Provide guidance on post-massage care, such as avoiding heavy meals, maintaining hydration, and refraining from vigorous exercise immediately after the session. This ensures that the benefits of the massage are maximized.

By following this step-by-step guide, practitioners can conduct a comprehensive and effective lymphatic drainage massage. The combination of face and body techniques contributes to a holistic approach that addresses both aesthetic and wellness concerns, promoting optimal lymphatic function and overall well-being.

5

TARGETING SPECIFIC SKIN CONCERNS

Addressing specific skin concerns is a key aspect of tailoring lymphatic drainage massage to individual needs. This section will delve into two common concerns: reducing puffiness and swelling, and improving circulation for a healthy glow. These targeted approaches highlight the versatility and effectiveness of lymphatic drainage massage in promoting skin health.

Reducing Puffiness and Swelling

Puffiness and swelling in various areas of the body, particularly the face, are common aesthetic concerns that can be effectively addressed through targeted lymphatic drainage massage techniques.

Facial Techniques:

1. Under-Eye Tapping:

Begin with gentle tapping or pulsing motions under the eyes. This technique stimulates lymphatic flow, reducing fluid retention that contributes to under-eye puffiness. Use the pads of the fingertips to tap lightly from the inner corners of the eyes towards the temples.

2. Jawline Sculpting:

Focus on the jawline to address facial bloating. Use upward and outward strokes along the jaw to guide excess fluid towards the lymph nodes. This helps define the contours of the face and reduces the appearance of a swollen or puffy jawline.

3. Nasolabial Fold Attention:

Pay special attention to the nasolabial fold area – the lines from the nose to the mouth. Utilize upward and outward strokes to encourage lymphatic drainage and diminish puffiness in this region.

Body Techniques:

1. Arm Elevation and Stroking:

Incorporate arm elevation during the massage to facilitate drainage. Position the arm slightly above heart level and use gentle, upward strokes towards the armpit. This helps reduce swelling in the arms and hands.

2. Leg Elevation and Circulation Movements:

Elevate the legs during the massage to aid in reducing swelling. Employ circular and upward strokes along the legs, directing fluid towards the lymph nodes in the groin. This is particularly beneficial for individuals dealing with leg swelling or edema.

3. Abdominal Techniques for Bloating:

Address abdominal bloating by incorporating specific techniques in this area. Use light, circular motions in a clockwise direction to support digestive function and reduce fluid retention in the abdomen.

The key to reducing puffiness and swelling lies in the precision and consistency of the massage techniques. By systematically targeting areas prone to fluid retention and utilizing gentle yet effective movements, lymphatic drainage massage offers a non-invasive and natural solution for individuals seeking to alleviate these specific skin concerns.

Improving Circulation for a Healthy Glow

Enhancing circulation is a fundamental goal of lymphatic drainage massage, contributing to a healthy glow and radiant complexion. Improved blood flow ensures that skin cells receive an ample supply of oxygen and nutrients, promoting overall skin health.

Facial Techniques:

1. Cheek and Forehead Stimulation:

Focus on the cheeks and forehead with light, sweeping motions. This helps boost blood circulation to these areas, imparting a rosy and vibrant complexion.

The increased circulation also contributes to a smoother and more even skin tone.

2. Under-Eye Revitalization:

Target the under-eye area with gentle tapping and pulsing motions. Improved circulation in this delicate region reduces dark circles and enhances the overall brightness of the eyes. Use the pads of the fingertips to stimulate blood flow and rejuvenate the under-eye skin.

3. Scalp Massage for Oxygenation:

Include a scalp massage to enhance oxygenation. Circular motions on the scalp stimulate blood flow, promoting the delivery of oxygen to the hair follicles and surrounding skin. This not only contributes to a healthy scalp but also adds to the overall glow of the face.

Body Techniques:

1. Upper Body Elevation:

Elevate the upper body during the massage to facilitate blood circulation. This is particularly beneficial for individuals dealing with issues like facial dullness or lack of radiance. Combine elevation with gentle strokes towards the heart to optimize circulation.

2. Leg Revitalization:

Use upward strokes along the legs to enhance blood flow. This technique is effective in reducing the appearance of cellulite and promoting a healthy, toned appearance. Improved circulation in the legs also supports overall skin vitality.

3. Abdominal Techniques for Digestive Health:

Incorporate techniques on the abdomen to support digestive health. Improved digestion contributes to better nutrient absorption, positively impacting the skin's radiance. Use gentle, clockwise circular motions to aid in the digestive process.

By focusing on techniques that specifically address circulation, lymphatic drainage massage becomes a holistic approach to achieving a healthy glow. The benefits extend beyond aesthetic improvements, encompassing the overall well-being of the skin. As blood circulation is optimized, the skin receives the nourishment it needs to thrive, resulting in a complexion that exudes vitality and radiance.

In conclusion, lymphatic drainage massage offers a versatile and targeted approach to addressing specific skin concerns. Whether it's reducing puffiness and swelling or enhancing circulation for a healthy glow, the precision and adaptability of this massage technique make it a valuable tool for individuals seeking both aesthetic and wellness benefits.

6

INTEGRATING ESSENTIAL OILS AND AROMATHERAPY

The integration of essential oils and aromatherapy into lymphatic drainage massage enhances not only the physical benefits but also the overall massage experience. This section will delve into the ways in which essential oils can elevate the massage experience and provide insights into the best oils for promoting skin health.

Enhancing the Massage Experience

Aromatherapy, the practice of using essential oils derived from plants for therapeutic purposes, adds a sensory dimension to the lymphatic drainage massage experience. The inhalation of aromatic compounds triggers responses in the brain that can influence mood, emotions, and even physiological functions. When combined with the gentle and rhythmic movements of lymphatic drainage massage, the synergy creates a holistic and immersive experience for the recipient.

Incorporating Essential Oils:

1. Lavender for Relaxation:

Lavender essential oil is renowned for its calming properties. Adding a few drops to the massage oil or diffusing it in the room can create a serene atmosphere, promoting relaxation and reducing stress levels. This is especially beneficial for individuals seeking not only physical benefits but also a mental and emotional reprieve.

2. Citrus Oils for Upliftment:

Citrus oils such as sweet orange or grapefruit are invigorating and uplifting. Their bright and citrusy scents can enhance the overall mood during the massage, providing a refreshing and energizing experience. These oils are particularly suitable for morning or daytime sessions.

3. Eucalyptus for Respiratory Support:

Eucalyptus essential oil has respiratory benefits and can be beneficial for individuals seeking additional respiratory support. Its invigorating scent can help clear the airways, promoting a sense of clarity and ease during the massage. This is especially relevant for those dealing with congestion or respiratory issues.

4. Chamomile for Soothing:

Chamomile essential oil is known for its soothing and anti-inflammatory properties. When incorporated into the massage, it can contribute to a calming effect on the skin and help reduce redness or irritation. This is ideal for individuals with sensitive skin or those looking to enhance the soothing aspect of the massage.

Application Techniques:

1. Diffusion in the Room:

Use an essential oil diffuser in the massage room to disperse the chosen essential oil into the air. This creates a subtle and consistent aroma, enveloping the client in a therapeutic atmosphere from the beginning to the end of the session.

2. Dilution in Massage Oil:

Blend a few drops of the selected essential oil into the massage oil or carrier oil. This ensures that the aroma is directly applied to the skin during the massage, providing both olfactory and topical benefits. Ensure that the chosen essential oil is safe for skin application and properly diluted.

3. Hot Towel Infusion:

Enhance the sensory experience by using hot towels infused with essential oils. Place a hot towel over specific areas of the body before or after the massage, allowing the soothing aroma to envelop the client and deepen the relaxation effect.

By integrating essential oils into lymphatic drainage massage, practitioners create a multisensory experience that goes beyond the physical manipulations of the massage techniques. The carefully selected aromas contribute to a personalized and immersive journey that caters to the individual's preferences and wellness goals.

Best Oils for Skin Health

In addition to enhancing the massage experience, the choice of essential oils can have specific benefits for skin health. Certain oils possess properties that align with the goals of lymphatic drainage massage, contributing to improved skin texture, hydration, and overall well-being.

Top Essential Oils for Skin Health:

1. Rosehip Seed Oil:

Renowned for its regenerative properties, rosehip seed oil is rich in vitamins and antioxidants. When integrated into lymphatic drainage massage, it promotes skin elasticity, reduces the appearance of scars and fine lines, and contributes to a radiant complexion.

2. Jojoba Oil:

Jojoba oil closely resembles the skin's natural sebum, making it an excellent choice for all skin types. It absorbs easily without clogging pores, providing hydration and balancing the skin's oil production. In lymphatic drainage massage, jojoba oil supports skin health without causing greasiness.

3. Grapeseed Oil:

Grapeseed oil is light and non-comedogenic, making it suitable for massage on the face and body. Rich in antioxidants, it helps protect the skin from free radicals and supports collagen production. The oil's quick absorption makes it an ideal carrier for essential oils during lymphatic drainage massage.

4. Calendula Oil:

Calendula oil is known for its anti-inflammatory and soothing properties. It can be beneficial for individuals with sensitive or irritated skin. When incorporated into lymphatic drainage massage, calendula oil helps calm the skin, reducing redness and promoting a balanced complexion.

Blending Techniques:

1. Customized Blends:

Tailor the massage oil by blending different essential oils and carrier oils to address specific skin concerns. For example, combining rosehip seed oil with a few drops of lavender essential oil creates a blend that nourishes the skin and promotes relaxation.

2. Hydrating Infusions:

Infuse massage oils with hydrating essential oils like chamomile or geranium. This enhances the moisturizing effect of the massage, leaving the skin supple and hydrated. This is particularly beneficial for individuals with dry or dehydrated skin.

3. Antioxidant-Rich Combinations:

Create blends that combine antioxidant-rich oils like grapeseed oil with uplifting essential oils such as citrus oils. This combination supports skin health by protecting against environmental stressors while providing a sensory boost during the massage.

Choosing the right essential oils and carrier oils for lymphatic drainage massage is a thoughtful and individualized process. The practitioner's expertise in selecting oils that align with the client's skin type, preferences, and desired outcomes ensures a tailored and effective massage experience.

In conclusion, integrating essential oils and aromatherapy into lymphatic drainage massage enhances both the physical and sensory aspects of the session. The careful selection and application of essential oils contribute to a holistic and personalized experience that addresses individual skin concerns

and elevates the overall well-being of the
client.

7

SELF-MASSAGE TECHNIQUES FOR HOMECARE

Self-massage techniques for homecare empower individuals to actively participate in their skincare routines, promoting skin maintenance, relaxation, and overall well-being. This section will delve into the importance of daily routines for skin maintenance and provide tips for effective self-massage.

Daily Routines for Skin Maintenance

Establishing a daily self-massage routine is a proactive and nurturing approach to maintaining skin health. Consistency is key, and dedicating a few minutes each day to self-massage can yield long-term benefits for the skin's appearance and overall well-being.

Morning Routine:

1. Facial Wake-Up Massage:

Begin the day with a gentle facial massage to awaken the skin. Use upward and outward strokes, focusing on the forehead, cheeks, and jawline. This helps stimulate blood circulation, reduce morning puffiness, and prepare the skin for the day ahead.

2. Neck and Shoulder Release:

Incorporate neck and shoulder massage to release tension. The neck and shoulder area often holds stress and stiffness. Use circular motions and gentle stretches to ease tension and promote relaxation. This not only benefits the skin but also contributes to a more relaxed overall state.

3. Arm and Hand Revitalization:

Extend the massage to the arms and hands. Utilize upward strokes towards the armpits and include circular motions on the hands and fingers. This boosts circulation, reduces stiffness, and supports fluid drainage.

Evening Routine:

1. Gentle Facial Cleanse and Massage:

Begin the evening routine with a gentle facial cleanse. Follow this with a calming facial massage using a hydrating oil or moisturizer. Focus on gentle strokes to relax facial muscles and promote a sense of tranquility before bedtime.

2. Relaxing Neck and Shoulder Massage:

Revisit the neck and shoulder area with a relaxing massage. Use slow and deliberate strokes to release accumulated tension from the day. This not only benefits the skin but also contributes to a restful night's sleep.

3. Leg and Foot Massage:

Conclude the evening routine with a soothing leg and foot massage. This can be particularly beneficial for individuals who spend long hours on their feet. Use upward strokes on the legs and include circular motions on the soles of the feet to relax and rejuvenate.

Tips for Effective Self-Massage

Ensuring that self-massage is both effective and enjoyable requires attention to technique, tools, and mindfulness. The following tips provide guidance for individuals seeking to enhance their self-massage practice:

1. Create a Relaxing Environment:

Set the stage for a positive self-massage experience by creating a calming environment. Dim the lights, play soothing music, and consider using aromatherapy through essential oils or candles to enhance relaxation.

2. Use the Right Tools:

Incorporate massage tools such as facial rollers, gua sha tools, or self-massage balls for specific areas. These tools can enhance the effectiveness of the massage and provide targeted relief.

3. Focus on Pressure and Speed:

Adjust the pressure and speed of your self-massage based on comfort and desired outcomes. For relaxation, use slow and gentle strokes, while firmer pressure may be suitable for areas with tension or tightness.

4. Pay Attention to Breathing:

Incorporate mindful breathing into your self-massage routine. Deep, slow breaths can enhance relaxation and help release tension. Sync your breath with the rhythm of your massage movements.

5. Tailor Techniques to Specific Areas:

Customize your self-massage techniques based on specific areas of concern. For example, use upward strokes on the face to counteract sagging, or focus on circular motions on the abdomen for digestive support.

6. Be Consistent:

Establish a consistent self-massage routine. Consistency is key for experiencing long-term benefits. Set aside dedicated time each day for self-massage, making it a cherished part of your self-care routine.

7. Incorporate Stretching:

Integrate stretching into your self-massage routine to enhance flexibility and release tension. Combining self-massage with gentle stretches can create a more comprehensive and rejuvenating experience.

8. Practice Mindfulness:

Approach self-massage with mindfulness. Be present in the moment, focusing on the sensations and the connection between your hands and the skin. Mindful self-massage can be a form of meditation, promoting mental clarity and relaxation.

9. Choose Suitable Products:

Select skincare products or oils that align with your skin type and goals. Whether you're focusing on hydration, anti-aging, or calming, choosing the right products enhances the effectiveness of the massage.

10. Listen to Your Body:

Pay attention to your body's signals during self-massage. If a particular area feels tender or sensitive, adjust the pressure accordingly. Listen to what your body needs and respond with care.

Self-massage techniques for homecare are not only about physical benefits but also about fostering a deeper connection with oneself. As you become attuned to your body's responses and engage in a mindful self-massage practice, the ritual becomes a holistic endeavor that supports both your physical and mental well-being.

11. Explore Different Techniques:

Don't hesitate to explore various self-massage techniques. From kneading and rolling motions to tapping or acupressure points, experimenting with different approaches can help you discover what feels most beneficial for your body.

12. Incorporate Facial Exercises:

Combine facial exercises with your self-massage routine. Gentle facial exercises, such as smiling widely or puffing out your cheeks, can complement the massage by toning facial muscles and promoting a youthful appearance.

13. Extend to Scalp Massage:

Include scalp massage in your routine for an additional dimension of relaxation. Use your fingertips to gently massage your scalp in circular motions. This not only promotes blood flow to the scalp but can also alleviate tension and stress.

14. Seek Professional Guidance:

Consider seeking guidance from a professional massage therapist or esthetician for personalized advice on self-massage techniques. They can provide insights into specific concerns or areas that may benefit from targeted attention.

15. Mind-Body Connection:

Foster a mind-body connection during your self-massage. As you touch and nurture your skin, cultivate a sense of gratitude for your body. This mindfulness can contribute to a positive self-image and a deeper appreciation for your body's resilience.

16. Utilize Online Resources:

Take advantage of online resources, such as video tutorials or guided self-massage sessions. Many practitioners share valuable insights and techniques that you can incorporate into your homecare routine. Follow trusted sources for reliable guidance.

17. Adapt to Your Schedule:

Recognize that your self-massage routine may need to adapt to your schedule. Whether you have a few minutes in the morning or prefer a longer session in the evening, tailor your routine to fit seamlessly into your daily life.

18. Combine with Skincare Rituals:

Integrate self-massage with your existing skincare rituals. Applying serums, moisturizers, or oils during the massage can enhance product absorption and maximize their benefits for your skin.

19. Address Specific Concerns:

If you have specific skin concerns, tailor your self-massage routine to address them. For example, focus on techniques that promote lymphatic drainage for reducing puffiness or incorporate gentle movements for areas prone to fine lines.

20. Embrace the Journey:

Embrace the journey of self-massage as a form of self-care and self-love. Allow the process to be nurturing and enjoyable, recognizing that this practice is a gift to yourself.

In conclusion, self-massage techniques for homecare extend beyond skincare—they encompass a holistic approach to well-being. By incorporating daily routines, utilizing effective techniques, and fostering mindfulness, individuals can experience the transformative power of self-massage.

This practice not only enhances skin health but also becomes a ritual of self-care, promoting a harmonious connection between the physical body and the nurturing touch of self-love.

8

COMBINING LYMPHATIC DRAINAGE WITH SKINCARE ROUTINE

The combination of lymphatic drainage massage with a tailored skincare routine creates a synergistic approach to achieving optimal skin health. This section will explore the importance of choosing the right skincare products and how to enhance results through proper skincare when incorporating lymphatic drainage massage.

Choosing the Right Skincare Products

Selecting the right skincare products is a foundational step in optimizing the benefits of lymphatic drainage massage. The synergy between effective products and massage techniques can address specific concerns, promote skin health, and contribute to a radiant complexion.

1. Cleansers:

Choose a gentle cleanser suitable for your skin type. Whether you have oily, dry, combination, or sensitive skin, a cleanser that removes impurities without stripping the skin's natural oils is crucial. Cleansing before a lymphatic drainage massage ensures a clean canvas for the massage techniques to be more effective.

2. Moisturizers:

Opt for a moisturizer that aligns with your skin's needs. Hydrating the skin is essential, and the right moisturizer can support the massage by enhancing glide and providing nourishment. Consider lightweight formulas for daytime use and richer options for nighttime hydration.

3. Serums:

Incorporate serums that target specific skin concerns. Whether you're addressing fine lines, uneven skin tone, or lack of radiance, serums with active ingredients can complement the effects of lymphatic drainage massage. Look for ingredients like vitamin C, hyaluronic acid, or peptides for added benefits.

4. Sunscreen:

Prioritize sunscreen as a non-negotiable step in your skincare routine. Sun protection is crucial for maintaining skin health and preventing premature aging. Apply sunscreen generously, especially if you've just undergone lymphatic drainage massage, as your skin may be more sensitive.

5. Eye Creams:

Choose an eye cream that addresses your specific concerns, such as puffiness, dark circles, or fine lines. Gentle massage techniques during lymphatic drainage can be enhanced by the application of an eye cream, contributing to a refreshed and revitalized eye area.

6. Targeted Treatments:

Consider incorporating targeted treatments based on your individual skin needs. This may include acne spot treatments, anti-aging creams, or products formulated to address hyperpigmentation. The combination of these treatments with lymphatic drainage massage can yield more noticeable and tailored results.

7. Natural and Organic Options:

If you prefer natural or organic skincare, explore products with clean formulations. Many natural ingredients, such as aloe vera, chamomile, or calendula, can complement the soothing effects of lymphatic drainage massage.

8. Consultation with Skincare Professionals:

Seek advice from skincare professionals or dermatologists for personalized product recommendations. A skincare professional can assess your skin type, concerns, and goals, providing insights into products that align with your unique needs.

Enhancing Results with Proper Skincare

Once you've chosen the right skincare products, the next step is to incorporate them effectively into your lymphatic drainage massage routine. Proper skincare enhances the massage experience, promotes skin health, and ensures long-term benefits.

1. Cleanse Before Massage:

Begin your lymphatic drainage massage routine with a clean face. Gently cleanse your skin to remove any makeup, impurities, or excess oils. This prepares the skin for the massage and allows the products applied during the routine to be more effectively absorbed.

2. Hydrate the Skin:

Apply a lightweight, hydrating product or facial mist before the massage. Hydrated skin allows for smoother movements during massage, enhancing the effectiveness of lymphatic drainage techniques. Consider using a hydrating toner or mist to prep the skin.

3. Incorporate Serums:

During the massage, use serums with active ingredients that cater to your skin concerns. The massage techniques facilitate better absorption of the serum, allowing the active ingredients to penetrate the skin more effectively. This synergy maximizes the benefits of both the massage and the skincare product.

4. Use Massage-Friendly Moisturizers:

Choose a moisturizer that complements the massage process. Lightweight, non-greasy formulas are ideal for daytime use, while richer creams can be incorporated into the evening routine. Applying a moisturizer after the massage helps seal in hydration and supports the skin's barrier function.

5. Eye Cream Application:

Apply your chosen eye cream during the massage, focusing on gentle tapping or rolling motions around the eye area. The massage enhances circulation, allowing the eye cream to penetrate the delicate skin, reducing puffiness and contributing to a more awake appearance.

6. Sunscreen After Morning Routine:

If you're performing lymphatic drainage massage in the morning, finish your routine with the application of sunscreen. Sun protection is paramount, especially when the skin may be more sensitive after massage. Choose a broad-spectrum sunscreen with adequate SPF for daily use.

7. Tailor Products to Massage Techniques:

Consider how the massage techniques align with the products you're using. For example, if you're focusing on lymphatic drainage for depuffing, choose products with soothing and anti-inflammatory ingredients to enhance the massage's calming effects.

8. Post-Massage Rehydration:

After completing the massage, rehydrate the skin with a refreshing mist or additional layer of lightweight moisturizer. This final step ensures that the skin remains nourished and supple post-massage.

9. Regularly Reassess Your Skincare Routine:

As your skin evolves, so should your skincare routine. Regularly reassess your products, adjusting them based on changes in your skin's needs or any specific concerns you may be addressing through lymphatic drainage massage.

10. Listen to Your Skin:

Pay attention to how your skin responds to the combination of lymphatic drainage massage and your skincare routine. If you notice positive changes or specific improvements, continue with the routine. Conversely, if your skin exhibits signs of sensitivity, reassess and potentially modify your approach.

11. Consider Professional Treatments:

Integrate professional skincare treatments, such as facials or professional lymphatic drainage massage sessions, into your routine periodically. Professional treatments can complement your at-home routine, providing deeper exfoliation, extraction, or specialized massage techniques for enhanced results.

Combining lymphatic drainage massage with a thoughtfully curated skincare routine transforms the daily ritual into a holistic and effective self-care practice. The synchronization of targeted products with specialized massage techniques supports skin health, addresses specific concerns, and contributes to a radiant complexion. As you embark on this integrated approach, remember that consistency and mindfulness are key elements in achieving lasting results and fostering a deep connection with your skin.

9

CLIENT SUCCESS STORIES

Client success stories are powerful narratives that showcase the tangible impact of lymphatic drainage massage on individuals' lives. These stories provide insights into real-life experiences and testimonials, offering a glimpse into the transformative effects of incorporating this massage technique into a wellness and skincare routine.

Real-life Experiences and Transformations

1. Reduction in Facial Puffiness and Improved Contouring:

Emma's Story

Emma, a 42-year-old professional, had been struggling with facial puffiness, particularly around her eyes and jawline. Concerned about the impact on her overall appearance, she decided to explore lymphatic drainage massage. After consistent sessions, Emma noticed a significant reduction in puffiness and improved facial contouring. The gentle techniques employed during the massage contributed to a more defined jawline and a revitalized appearance, boosting Emma's confidence.

2. Alleviation of Chronic Headaches and Tension:

David's Journey

David, a 35-year-old with a high-stress job, experienced chronic headaches and tension in his neck and shoulders. Seeking a holistic solution, he integrated lymphatic drainage massage into his self-care routine. Over time, David reported a remarkable alleviation of his headaches and tension. The combination of massage techniques targeting the neck and shoulder area, along with the calming effects of the sessions, brought about a transformative change in David's overall well-being.

3.Post-Surgery Recovery and Scar Healing:

Sarah's Testimonial

Sarah underwent surgery that left her with visible scars. Eager to support her body's healing process, she incorporated lymphatic drainage massage into her recovery plan. Through targeted techniques on and around the scar tissue, Sarah witnessed not only accelerated healing but also a reduction in scar visibility. The massage played a vital role in enhancing circulation, promoting lymphatic drainage, and contributing to Sarah's positive post-surgery outcome.

4. Enhanced Skin Radiance and Vibrancy:

Michael's Experience

Michael, a 50-year-old fitness enthusiast, was seeking ways to enhance his skin's radiance. Intrigued by the benefits of lymphatic drainage massage, he decided to give it a try. The results surpassed his expectations—Michael noticed a vibrant and healthy glow to his skin after consistent sessions. The improved circulation and detoxification brought about by the massage techniques had a transformative effect on Michael's skin, reflecting his dedication to overall well-being.

Testimonials Highlighting Holistic Well-being

1. Stress Reduction and Improved Sleep Quality:

Julia's Testimonial

Julia, a busy mother of two, struggled with stress and difficulty falling asleep. Seeking a natural approach, she integrated lymphatic drainage massage into her bedtime routine. The calming effects of the massage not only reduced Julia's stress levels but also contributed to improved sleep quality. Julia's testimonial reflects the holistic impact of the massage on both her physical and mental well-being.

2. Digestive Support and Alleviation of Bloating:

Alex's Journey

Alex, a 28-year-old with occasional digestive issues, explored lymphatic drainage massage as a complementary approach to support his digestive health. The massage techniques targeting the abdominal area played a significant role in alleviating bloating and promoting healthy digestion. Alex's success story highlights the interconnectedness of lymphatic drainage massage and overall digestive well-being.

3. Boosted Immune Function and Reduced Seasonal Allergies:

Sophie's Success

Sophie, who experienced seasonal allergies, decided to explore alternative methods to support her immune system.

Incorporating lymphatic drainage massage into her routine resulted in a notable reduction in allergy symptoms. The massage's ability to stimulate lymphatic flow contributed to a strengthened immune function, providing Sophie with relief from the challenges of seasonal allergies.

4. Emotional Healing and Mindful Self-Care:

Mark's Transformation

Mark, navigating a period of emotional upheaval, turned to lymphatic drainage massage as a form of mindful self-care. The calming and grounding nature of the massage provided Mark with not only physical relaxation but also emotional healing. His testimonial emphasizes the holistic benefits of incorporating lymphatic drainage into a self-care routine during challenging times.

Common Themes in Client Success Stories

1. Holistic Wellness:

Across various success stories, a common theme emerges—lymphatic drainage massage contributes to holistic wellness. Clients frequently report improvements not only in specific skin concerns but also in overall physical and mental well-being. This highlights the interconnected nature of the lymphatic system and its impact on various aspects of health.

2. Tailored Approaches:

Each success story reflects a tailored approach to addressing individual concerns. Whether it's reducing puffiness, supporting post-surgery recovery, or enhancing skin vibrancy, the versatility of lymphatic drainage massage allows for personalized and targeted interventions.

3. Consistency and Commitment:

Successful outcomes are often linked to consistency and commitment. Clients who incorporate lymphatic drainage massage into their routines and make it a regular part of their self-care practices tend to experience more significant and lasting benefits. The commitment to regular sessions reflects an understanding of the cumulative effects of lymphatic drainage massage on the body's natural processes.

4. Integrative Wellness Practices:

Client success stories frequently highlight the integration of lymphatic drainage massage into a broader wellness framework. This may include a combination of healthy lifestyle choices, skincare routines, and other holistic practices. The holistic approach emphasizes that optimal well-being is a multifaceted journey that extends beyond individual interventions.

5. Emotional and Mental Well-being:

Beyond physical benefits, several success stories emphasize the positive impact of lymphatic drainage massage on emotional and mental well-being. The calming and grounding effects of the massage contribute to stress reduction, improved sleep quality, and emotional healing. This holistic approach aligns with the growing recognition of the mind-body connection in overall health.

6. Empowerment through Self-Care:

Many clients express a sense of empowerment through their journey with lymphatic drainage massage. By actively participating in their self-care routines, individuals feel a renewed sense of control over their well-being. This empowerment extends beyond the massage sessions, influencing other aspects of their lives.

7. Supportive Role in Recovery:

Success stories related to post-surgery recovery highlight the supportive role of lymphatic drainage massage in healing processes. Clients report not only accelerated recovery but also reduced discomfort and improved scar healing. These testimonials underscore the potential of lymphatic drainage massage as a complementary approach to traditional medical interventions.

8. Enhanced Self-Image and Confidence:

Several success stories touch upon the positive impact of lymphatic drainage massage on individuals' self-image and confidence. Whether addressing concerns related to facial appearance or supporting overall skin health, clients often report feeling more confident and comfortable in their own skin after incorporating lymphatic drainage into their routines.

Sharing Success Stories for Inspiration

Sharing these success stories not only serves as a testament to the efficacy of lymphatic drainage massage but also provides inspiration for others considering or undergoing similar wellness journeys. Real-life experiences and testimonials create a sense of relatability, offering hope and encouragement to those seeking solutions for their specific concerns.

1. Community Support and Connection:

As success stories are shared within communities, whether online or through wellness centers, a sense of support and connection emerges. Individuals facing similar challenges find solace in knowing that others have navigated similar paths and achieved positive outcomes through lymphatic drainage massage.

2. Education and Awareness:

Success stories play a crucial role in educating individuals about the benefits of lymphatic drainage massage. They contribute to raising awareness about the diverse applications of this technique, from skincare enhancements to broader wellness benefits. Through firsthand accounts, potential clients gain insights into what they can expect and how lymphatic drainage may align with their goals.

3.   Motivation   for   Personal Transformation:

Personal transformation often begins with inspiration. Success stories serve as motivational   tools,   encouraging individuals to embark on their own wellness   journeys.   The   relatable narratives create a bridge between the potential for positive change and the actionable steps individuals can take to achieve their desired outcomes.

4. Building Trust in the Practice:

For those new to lymphatic drainage massage, success stories play a pivotal role in building trust in the practice. Real-life experiences from others who have witnessed tangible improvements instill confidence in the effectiveness and safety of the massage techniques. Trust is a crucial component of any wellness practice, and success stories contribute to its establishment.

5. Fostering a Positive Outlook:

Success stories contribute to fostering a positive outlook on wellness. As individuals share their journeys of overcoming challenges and achieving positive results, a collective narrative emerges—one that emphasizes the potential for improvement, rejuvenation, and overall well-being through the integration of lymphatic drainage massage.

In conclusion, client success stories offer a rich tapestry of experiences, showcasing the multifaceted benefits of lymphatic drainage massage. From physical transformations to emotional healing and empowerment, these narratives inspire and inform individuals on their own wellness journeys. By sharing these stories within communities and amplifying awareness, the positive impact of lymphatic drainage massage continues to unfold, creating a supportive and inspiring environment for those seeking to enhance their well-being.

FAQS ABOUT LYMPHATIC DRAINAGE MASSAGE

Lymphatic drainage massage is a specialized technique that focuses on stimulating the lymphatic system, aiming to improve lymph circulation and promote overall well-being. Here are answers to some commonly asked questions about this therapeutic practice:

1. What is Lymphatic Drainage Massage, and how does it work?

Lymphatic drainage massage is a therapeutic technique designed to stimulate the lymphatic system, a crucial component of the body's immune system. The lymphatic system helps eliminate toxins, waste, and excess fluid from the body. The massage involves gentle, rhythmic strokes and movements, aimed at encouraging the flow of lymphatic fluid. By promoting lymph circulation, the massage supports the body's natural detoxification process and enhances immune function.

2. What are the Benefits of Lymphatic Drainage Massage for the Skin?

Lymphatic drainage massage offers various benefits for the skin, including:

- Reduced Puffiness: The massage helps to reduce fluid retention and puffiness, particularly in the face and eyes.
- Improved Radiance: By enhancing lymph circulation, the massage promotes a healthy glow and radiant complexion.
- Detoxification: It aids in removing toxins and waste products from the skin, contributing to clearer and healthier skin.

- Enhanced Texture: Regular lymphatic drainage can improve skin texture by reducing inflammation and promoting tissue regeneration.

3. Is Lymphatic Drainage Massage Painful?

Lymphatic drainage massage is generally not painful. The techniques involve gentle, rhythmic movements that aim to stimulate lymph flow without causing discomfort. Clients may experience a sensation of light pressure, but it should not be painful. If you have specific concerns or areas of sensitivity, it's essential to communicate with your massage therapist, who can adjust the pressure accordingly.

4. How Long Does a Lymphatic Drainage Massage Session Typically Last?

The duration of a lymphatic drainage massage session can vary but typically lasts between 60 to 90 minutes. The therapist will assess your individual needs and goals to determine the appropriate session length. Longer sessions may be recommended for individuals with specific health concerns or those seeking a more comprehensive lymphatic support.

5. Can Lymphatic Drainage Massage Help with Post-Surgery Recovery?

Yes, lymphatic drainage massage is often recommended for post-surgery recovery. The gentle techniques can aid in reducing swelling, promoting the removal of excess fluid, and supporting overall healing. It's crucial to consult with your healthcare provider and seek the expertise of a qualified massage therapist who has experience in post-surgery recovery massage.

6. Are There Any Contraindications for Lymphatic Drainage Massage?

While lymphatic drainage massage is generally safe for most individuals, there are some contraindications and precautions to consider. Contraindications may include acute infections, certain cancers, congestive heart failure, and acute thrombosis. It's essential to inform your massage therapist about any pre-existing health conditions or concerns to ensure the massage is tailored to your specific needs.

7. How Often Should I Get Lymphatic Drainage Massage?

The frequency of lymphatic drainage massage depends on individual goals and health considerations. For general well-being and maintenance, monthly sessions may be sufficient. However, individuals undergoing post-surgery recovery or addressing specific health concerns may benefit from more frequent sessions initially. The frequency can be discussed and determined in consultation with a qualified massage therapist.

8. Can Lymphatic Drainage Massage Help with Cellulite Reduction?

Lymphatic drainage massage may contribute to cellulite reduction by promoting lymphatic circulation and fluid drainage. While it may not eliminate cellulite entirely, regular sessions can help improve the appearance of skin texture and reduce the fluid retention associated with cellulite. Combining lymphatic drainage with a healthy lifestyle, including hydration and exercise, can enhance results.

9. *Is Lymphatic Drainage Massage Suitable for Everyone?*

Lymphatic drainage massage is generally suitable for many individuals, but there are considerations based on individual health conditions. It's crucial to inform your massage therapist about any medical conditions, ongoing treatments, or concerns you may have. Pregnant individuals, those with certain medical conditions, or individuals on specific medications may need modifications to the massage techniques.

10. *Can I Perform Lymphatic Drainage Massage at Home?*

While self-massage techniques inspired by lymphatic drainage principles can be performed at home, professional lymphatic drainage massage involves specialized training. It's recommended to seek guidance from a qualified massage therapist or healthcare professional before attempting self-massage, especially if you have specific health concerns or are recovering from surgery.

11. How Soon Can I See Results from Lymphatic Drainage Massage?

The timing for noticeable results from lymphatic drainage massage varies based on individual factors, including health conditions, lifestyle, and the frequency of sessions. Some individuals may experience immediate improvements in reduced puffiness and enhanced skin radiance, while others may observe cumulative benefits over several sessions.

12. Can Lymphatic Drainage Massage Help with Sinus Congestion?

Yes, lymphatic drainage massage can be beneficial for sinus congestion. The techniques involved can help promote drainage of excess fluids, reduce inflammation, and alleviate pressure in the sinus areas. This can be particularly helpful for individuals experiencing sinus issues due to allergies, colds, or other respiratory conditions.

13. Are There Any Specific Preparations Before a Lymphatic Drainage Massage Session?

There are no specific preparations required before a lymphatic drainage massage session. However, it's advisable to communicate any health concerns, recent surgeries, or medications you are taking with your massage therapist. Wear comfortable clothing, as the therapist may need access to specific areas of your body. Additionally, staying hydrated before the session can enhance the effectiveness of the massage by promoting fluid movement in the lymphatic system.

14. Can Lymphatic Drainage Massage Help with Digestive Issues?

Yes, lymphatic drainage massage can provide support for digestive issues. The massage techniques, especially when applied to the abdominal area, can aid in promoting healthy digestion, reducing bloating, and supporting the overall function of the digestive system. However, it's essential to consult with your healthcare provider if you have specific digestive concerns.

15. Does Lymphatic Drainage Massage Require Specialized Training for Therapists?

Yes, lymphatic drainage massage requires specialized training for therapists. Professionals undergo specific training to learn the appropriate techniques that focus on stimulating the lymphatic system. It's crucial to seek out a qualified massage therapist who has received proper training and certification in lymphatic drainage massage to ensure a safe and effective session.

16. Can Lymphatic Drainage Massage Help with Weight Loss?

Lymphatic drainage massage is not a direct method for weight loss. While the massage can assist in reducing fluid retention and promoting detoxification, it does not lead to significant or permanent weight loss. It's important to approach lymphatic drainage massage as a supportive practice within a comprehensive wellness plan that includes a balanced diet and regular physical activity.

17. What Should I Expect During a Lymphatic Drainage Massage Session?

During a lymphatic drainage massage session, you can expect to lie comfortably on a massage table. The therapist will use gentle, rhythmic strokes and specific movements to stimulate the flow of lymphatic fluid. Sessions are generally relaxing, and clients often experience a sense of lightness and increased well-being afterward. Communication with the therapist is encouraged to ensure the session is tailored to your preferences and needs.

18. Are There Any Side Effects of Lymphatic Drainage Massage?

While lymphatic drainage massage is generally safe, some individuals may experience mild side effects. These can include increased urination, temporary changes in bowel movements, or a feeling of fatigue. These effects are usually transient and indicate the body's natural detoxification response. It's important to stay hydrated after a session to support the elimination of toxins.

19. Can Lymphatic Drainage Massage Be Combined with Other Massage Techniques?

Yes, lymphatic drainage massage can be combined with other massage techniques based on individual needs and preferences. Therapists may integrate elements of Swedish massage, deep tissue massage, or other modalities depending on the client's goals. Combining techniques allows for a customized approach that addresses specific concerns while providing overall relaxation.

20. Is Lymphatic Drainage Massage Safe for Pregnant Women?

Lymphatic drainage massage can be safe for pregnant women when performed by a qualified and experienced therapist who is knowledgeable about prenatal massage. The techniques are adapted to ensure the comfort and safety of the mother and baby. However, it's crucial to consult with a healthcare provider before scheduling a lymphatic drainage massage during pregnancy, especially for individuals with high-risk pregnancies or specific medical conditions.

21. How Can I Find a Qualified Lymphatic Drainage Massage Therapist?

To find a qualified lymphatic drainage massage therapist, consider the following steps:

- Check Credentials: Ensure that the therapist has proper certification and training in lymphatic drainage massage.
- Read Reviews: Look for reviews from previous clients to gauge the therapist's expertise and professionalism.
-Ask for Recommendations: Seek recommendations from healthcare providers, friends, or family members who may have had positive experiences with a specific therapist.

- Inquire about Experience: Choose a therapist with experience in addressing specific concerns or conditions relevant to your needs.

- Schedule a Consultation: Before booking a session, schedule a consultation to discuss your goals, health history, and any concerns you may have.

Choosing a qualified and reputable therapist is crucial to ensuring a safe and effective lymphatic drainage massage experience.

In conclusion, these FAQs provide comprehensive insights into various aspects of lymphatic drainage massage. Whether addressing common questions about the technique's benefits, safety, or integration with other wellness practices, understanding these aspects can help individuals make informed decisions about incorporating lymphatic drainage

massage into their overall well-being and
skincare routines.

CONCLUSION

Lymphatic drainage massage emerges as a transformative practice that extends beyond traditional massage techniques, offering a range of benefits for both physical and mental well-being. As we conclude our exploration, let's recap the key benefits and emphasize the importance of encouraging regular maintenance.

Recap of Benefits:

1. Improved Lymphatic Circulation: Lymphatic drainage massage serves as a gentle yet powerful method to stimulate the lymphatic system, promoting optimal circulation. This enhanced flow aids in the removal of toxins, waste, and excess fluid, contributing to overall detoxification.

2. Radiant and Healthy Skin: One of the standout benefits is the positive impact on skin health. The massage techniques help reduce puffiness, improve skin texture, and contribute to a radiant complexion. Clients often experience a visible glow as a result of improved lymphatic circulation.*

3. Post-Surgery Support: Lymphatic drainage massage plays a vital role in post-surgery recovery by reducing swelling, promoting healing, and supporting the body's natural processes. The gentle techniques provide comfort and aid in the restoration of optimal functioning.

4. Stress Reduction and Relaxation: Beyond its physical benefits, lymphatic drainage massage is known for its calming effects. The rhythmic

movements induce relaxation, alleviate tension, and contribute to an overall sense of well-being. This dual focus on both physical and mental aspects sets it apart as a holistic practice.

5. Digestive and Immune Support: The massage's impact extends to digestive health, helping with bloating and promoting a healthy digestive system. Additionally, by supporting lymphatic circulation, the practice contributes to a strengthened immune function, providing resilience against illnesses.

Encouraging Regular Maintenance:

As we reflect on the manifold benefits of lymphatic drainage massage, it becomes evident that regular maintenance is key to unlocking its full potential. Here are key points to consider:

1.   Consistency   Yields   Cumulative Benefits:

Regular sessions allow for the cumulative benefits of lymphatic drainage massage to manifest. The gentle yet persistent stimulation of the lymphatic system yields more noticeable and lasting results over time. Consistency is the cornerstone of reaping the rewards this practice has to offer.

2. Holistic Well-being Demands Ongoing Care:

Holistic well-being encompasses both physical and mental dimensions. Regular maintenance through lymphatic drainage massage aligns with the philosophy of nurturing the body and mind as an integrated system. Ongoing care fosters a harmonious balance that extends beyond momentary relief to sustained vitality.

3. Tailoring Sessions to Evolving Needs:

Regular maintenance allows for the tailoring of sessions to evolving needs. As individuals progress in their wellness journey, the focus of lymphatic drainage massage can be adjusted to address specific concerns. This adaptability ensures that the practice remains relevant and effective in supporting changing health goals.

4. Preemptive Wellness Investment:

Viewing lymphatic drainage massage as a preemptive wellness investment is a proactive approach. By incorporating regular sessions into one's routine, individuals invest in their long-term health. This preventative perspective aligns with a broader commitment to self-care and a proactive approach to well-being.

5. Integration with Skincare Rituals:

The integration of lymphatic drainage massage into skincare rituals further emphasizes the importance of regular maintenance. By combining this therapeutic practice with a consistent skincare routine, individuals create a comprehensive approach that addresses both the internal and external aspects of skin health.

6. Empowering Self-care Practices:

Regular maintenance through lymphatic drainage massage empowers individuals in their self-care journey. By actively participating in ongoing sessions, individuals take charge of their well-being, fostering a sense of agency and control over their health. This empowerment extends beyond the massage table into daily life.

7. Collaboration with Skincare Professionals:

Collaborating with skincare professionals and massage therapists ensures a personalized and informed approach to regular maintenance. These experts can provide guidance on session frequency, targeted techniques, and the integration of complementary practices, ensuring an optimized wellness plan.

8. Nurturing Mind-Body Connection:

Regular maintenance nurtures the mind-body connection. As individuals consistently engage in lymphatic drainage massage, they deepen their awareness of how physical well-being intertwines with mental and emotional states. This heightened consciousness contributes to a holistic understanding of self-care.

In conclusion, lymphatic drainage massage emerges not only as a therapeutic practice with diverse benefits but also as a pathway to ongoing well-being. Through regular maintenance, individuals embark on a journey of sustained health, embracing the transformative potential of this holistic practice. As the rhythm of gentle strokes continues, so does the symphony of well-being—a harmonious melody of vitality, radiance, and resilience.

GLOSSARY OF TERMS

In the realm of lymphatic drainage massage and holistic well-being, understanding the terminology associated with this practice is essential. Let's explore a comprehensive glossary that encompasses key terms, concepts, and techniques relevant to lymphatic drainage massage.

1. Lymphatic System:

The body's network of vessels, nodes, and organs that work together to transport lymph, a clear fluid containing white blood cells, throughout the body. The lymphatic system plays a crucial role in immune function, detoxification, and fluid balance.

2. Lymph Nodes:

Small, bean-shaped structures that filter and purify lymph as it travels through the lymphatic system. Lymph nodes contain immune cells that help combat infections and remove harmful substances.

3. Lymph:

The clear fluid that circulates through the lymphatic system, carrying white blood cells, proteins, and waste products. Lymph plays a vital role in immune response and maintaining fluid balance.

4. Lymphatic Drainage Massage:

A therapeutic massage technique designed to stimulate the lymphatic system, promoting lymph circulation, detoxification, and overall well-being. The massage involves gentle, rhythmic strokes aimed at encouraging the movement of lymphatic fluid.

5. Edema:

Swelling caused by the accumulation of excess fluid in body tissues. Lymphatic drainage massage is often used to reduce edema by promoting fluid movement and drainage.

6. Detoxification:

The process of eliminating toxins and waste products from the body. Lymphatic drainage massage supports detoxification by enhancing lymph circulation, allowing the removal of metabolic waste.

7. Contraindications:

Factors or conditions that make a particular treatment or intervention potentially harmful or inappropriate. In the context of lymphatic drainage massage, contraindications may include acute infections, certain cancers, or conditions that affect lymphatic flow.

8. Rhythmic Techniques:

Massage techniques characterized by a repetitive and flowing pattern. In lymphatic drainage massage, rhythmic techniques are employed to stimulate lymphatic flow gently.

9. Manual Lymphatic Mapping:

A technique used to assess the lymphatic system by manually mapping the flow of lymph in the body. This mapping guides therapists in tailoring the massage to address specific areas of concern.

10. Effleurage:

A massage stroke involving long, sweeping movements over the skin. In lymphatic drainage massage, effleurage helps initiate the gentle stimulation of lymphatic flow.

11. Compression Therapy:

A therapeutic technique that involves the application of pressure to specific areas of the body to promote circulation and reduce swelling. Compression garments may be used as part of lymphatic drainage therapy.

12. Post-Surgery Recovery Massage:

Lymphatic drainage massage applied to individuals recovering from surgery to reduce swelling, promote healing, and support the body's natural recovery processes.

13. Cellulite Reduction Massage:

Massage techniques targeting areas affected by cellulite to improve skin texture, promote circulation, and reduce fluid retention. While not a direct solution to cellulite, it can enhance the appearance of the skin.

14. Hydrotherapy:

The use of water in various forms (such as hot and cold applications, compresses, or baths) for therapeutic purposes. Hydrotherapy can complement lymphatic drainage massage by promoting circulation and relaxation.

15. Reflexology:

A complementary therapy that involves applying pressure to specific points on the hands, feet, or ears to stimulate corresponding areas of the body. Reflexology may be integrated with lymphatic drainage massage for enhanced well-being.

16. Manual Lymphatic Drainage (MLD):

A specialized form of massage focusing on gentle, specific movements to stimulate lymphatic flow. Manual Lymphatic Drainage is often used to address lymphedema, post-surgery recovery, and various health concerns.

17. Self-Massage Techniques:

Techniques individuals can perform on themselves to stimulate lymphatic flow. Self-massage may involve gentle strokes, circular movements, or tapping in specific areas to support lymphatic drainage.

18. Skincare Rituals:

Personalized routines that individuals follow to care for their skin. Lymphatic drainage massage can be integrated into skincare rituals to enhance skin health and radiance.

19. Aromatherapy:

The use of essential oils derived from plants to promote physical and psychological well-being. In lymphatic drainage massage, aromatherapy may be incorporated to enhance the overall massage experience.

20. Holistic Wellness:

A holistic approach to well-being considers the interconnectedness of physical, mental, and emotional health. Lymphatic drainage massage aligns with the principles of holistic wellness by addressing multiple facets of an individual's health.

21. Craniosacral Therapy:

A therapeutic modality involving gentle manipulation of the skull and spine to enhance the flow of cerebrospinal fluid. While distinct from lymphatic drainage massage, craniosacral therapy may be used in conjunction to support overall well-being.

22. Inflammation:

A natural response of the body to injury or infection, characterized by redness, swelling, pain, and heat. Lymphatic drainage massage aids in reducing inflammation by promoting the removal of inflammatory substances and supporting the body's healing processes.

23. Essential Oils:

Concentrated aromatic compounds extracted from plants that are used for their therapeutic properties. Essential oils may be integrated into lymphatic drainage massage for added relaxation, skin benefits, and overall enhancement of the massage experience.

24. Cupping Therapy:

A therapeutic technique involving the use of suction cups to create negative pressure on the skin. While not a direct part of lymphatic drainage massage, cupping therapy may be used in combination to address specific concerns such as muscle tension and circulation.

25. Acupressure:

A technique involving the application of pressure to specific points on the body to promote relaxation and balance energy flow. Acupressure points may be incorporated into lymphatic drainage massage for targeted benefits.

26. Therapeutic Grade:

Refers to essential oils that meet specific quality standards for purity and potency. When using essential oils in lymphatic drainage massage, choosing therapeutic-grade oils ensures a high-quality and safe experience.

27. Posture Assessment:

An evaluation of an individual's body posture to identify imbalances or misalignments. Posture assessment may be part of the client assessment process before a lymphatic drainage massage to tailor the session to specific needs.

28. Holistic Nutrition:

A nutritional approach that considers the whole person—physical, mental, and emotional aspects—in developing a balanced and individualized diet. Holistic nutrition can complement the benefits of lymphatic drainage massage by supporting overall health.

29. Hydration:

The act of maintaining adequate fluid levels in the body. Staying hydrated is crucial before and after lymphatic drainage massage to support the elimination of toxins and enhance overall well-being.

30. Homecare Routine:

A personalized routine individuals follow at home to support the benefits of lymphatic drainage massage. This may include self-massage, skincare practices, and other wellness activities.

31. Immunocompetence:

The ability of the immune system to effectively respond to and defend against infections and diseases. Lymphatic drainage massage supports immunocompetence by promoting lymph circulation and enhancing immune function.

32. Tension Headaches:

Headaches caused by muscle tension and stress. Lymphatic drainage massage can be beneficial in relieving tension headaches by promoting relaxation and reducing muscle tension.

33. Post-Event Massage:

Massage applied after physical activities or events to aid in recovery and reduce muscle soreness. Lymphatic drainage massage techniques may be incorporated into post-event massage for added benefits.

34. Hydrostatic Pressure:

The pressure exerted by a fluid, such as water, at rest. Hydrostatic pressure plays a role in lymphatic drainage by influencing fluid movement within the body.

35. Alleviation of Congestion:

The reduction or relief of blockages or buildup, particularly in the context of sinus or respiratory congestion. Lymphatic drainage massage can help alleviate congestion by promoting drainage and reducing fluid buildup.

36. Mind-Body Connection:

The interrelationship between mental and physical well-being. Lymphatic drainage massage contributes to the mind-body connection by promoting relaxation and reducing stress.

37. Chronic Fatigue Syndrome:

A complex disorder characterized by persistent, unexplained fatigue. Lymphatic drainage massage may be considered as part of a holistic approach to managing symptoms and supporting overall well-being.

38. Therapeutic Integration:

The incorporation of multiple therapeutic modalities into a comprehensive approach. Lymphatic drainage massage therapists may integrate various techniques to address specific client needs and goals.

39. Rebounding Exercise:

A form of low-impact exercise performed on a trampoline. Rebounding can be complementary to lymphatic drainage massage by promoting circulation and supporting lymphatic flow.

40. Mindful Self-Care:

The practice of consciously engaging in activities that promote well-being and self-awareness. Lymphatic drainage massage aligns with mindful self-care by fostering relaxation and encouraging individuals to be present in their well-being journey.

In conclusion, this glossary provides a comprehensive overview of terms related to lymphatic drainage massage and its integration with various therapeutic modalities. Understanding these terms enhances one's appreciation for the holistic nature of lymphatic drainage massage and its multifaceted impact on well-being.